LOVE
Thyself

EMPOWERING MEN FOR HEALTHY LIVING

I0106535

ANTONIO M. PALMER

LOVE THYSELF
Empowering Men For Healthy Living

Published by Kingdom Publishing LLC
Odenton, MD 21113

Printed in the U.S.A.

Copyright ©2025 by Antonio M. Palmer

All rights reserved. No part of this book may be reproduced, stored in retrieval system, or transmitted in any form or by any means—electronic, mechanical, photocopy, recording or otherwise—except for brief quotations in printed reviews, without the prior written permission of the author.

Unless otherwise indicated, all Scripture quotations are taken from the King James Version (KJV) of the Holy Bible which is public domain. Scripture quotations noted NIV are from the Holy Bible: New International Version® copyright ©1973, 1978, 1984 by International Bible Society. Used by permission of Zondervan Publishing House. All rights reserved.

ISBN: 978-1-947741-99-7

Table of Contents

— Dedicated —
*to all men who desire to grow and
be the man God created you to be.*

Introduction
Do You Want to be Made Whole?

In the Gospel of John, Jesus encounters a man by the pool of Bethesda who had been an invalid for thirty-eight years. In a moment of divine compassion and power, Jesus asks him, *"Do you want to be made whole?"* (John 5:6, KJV). This profound question transcends time, echoing into the hearts of humanity today. Jesus' healing of the man wasn't just about physical restoration—it was about bringing him into a state of total wholeness: body, mind, and soul. To be "made whole" in the biblical sense encompasses completeness, health, and harmony in every area of life. It is about living in alignment with God's purpose while thriving in the fullness of His blessings.

But how can we walk in this wholeness if we neglect the very vessel God has given us—ourselves? In Matthew 22:39, Jesus commands us to *"love your neighbor as yourself."* This statement implies that self-love is not just acceptable but essential. You cannot love others well if you do not first know how to love and care for yourself. True self-love is not selfishness; it is stewardship—managing what God has entrusted to you well.

This book, Love Thyself, explores the five critical dimensions of self-care: physical, spiritual, mental, financial, and domestic. Each dimension is interconnected, and neglecting one impacts the others. For example, financial stress can affect mental health, a cluttered home can drain energy, and poor physical health can hinder one's ability to fulfill one's spiritual purpose.

Through the pages of this book, we'll explore how to honor God by caring for yourself holistically. You'll discover practical strategies, biblical wisdom, and empowering truths to help you:

- Nurture your body as a temple of the Holy Spirit.
- Strengthen your spirit through faith, prayer, and worship.
- Cultivate a sound and peaceful mind.
- Manage your finances with integrity and wisdom.
- Create a domestic environment that fosters peace and joy.

Jesus came so that we might have life and have it more abundantly (John 10:10). Abundance begins with wholeness. When you learn to love yourself well, you position yourself to serve God and others more effectively, reflecting His glory in every facet of your life.

Are you ready to embrace the fullness of life that Jesus offers? Let's embark on this transformative journey together, learning to love ourselves the way God intended and answering His call to be made whole.

Chapter 1
The Man and His Body
Physical Health

"I wish above all things that you would prosper and be in health even as your soul prospers."
(3 John 2)

Your Health is Your Wealth!

The Power of Physical Health in Wholeness

Good health is one of the greatest treasures a man can possess. The phrase "Your health is your wealth" underscores the truth that without physical, mental, and emotional well-being, all other forms of success lose their value. In this chapter, we will explore how maintaining physical health contributes to living a life of wholeness and provides practical tools to help you build a foundation of health for yourself and your loved ones.

Why Physical Health Matters

1. Physical Health Fuels Productivity

    A healthy body empowers you to work, pursue your dreams, and engage in activities that bring joy and fulfillment. When health is neglected, limitations arise that hinder productivity and the ability to enjoy life's blessings.

2. Mental and Emotional Health Are Connected to Physical Health

    Emotional and mental resilience are essential aspects of wholeness. Stress, anxiety, and depression can take a toll on your physical health, just as poor physical health can affect your emotional well-being.

3. Wealth Cannot Replace Health

While money may purchase medical care, it cannot restore health once lost. Preventive care and intentional health-focused decisions are far more effective than trying to reverse years of neglect.

4. Good Health Brings Fulfillment

A vibrant, healthy life allows you to enjoy relationships, experiences, and achievements more fully. It creates the capacity for longevity, vitality, and happiness.

Men's Health Priorities

Maintaining physical health involves addressing specific challenges men face. Below are the top health risks for men and strategies to prevent them.

Top Health Risks for Men

1. Heart Disease
   - Cause: Poor diet, inactivity, high cholesterol, smoking. 21.6% of all deaths among African American men is caused by heart disease. It is also the leading cause of death among men worldwide.
   - Prevention: Exercise regularly, eat a heart-healthy diet, and manage blood pressure.

2. Cancer (Prostate, Lung, Colorectal)
   - Cause: Smoking, diet, and genetics.
   - Prevention: Get regular screenings and maintain a nutrient-dense diet.

3. Accidental Injuries
   - Cause: Distracted driving, workplace hazards.
   - Prevention: Wear seat belts, avoid distractions, and follow safety protocols.

4. Type 2 Diabetes
   - Cause: Obesity, poor diet, lack of exercise.
   - Prevention: Maintain a healthy weight and reduce sugar consumption.

5. Suicide and Mental Health Disorders
   - Cause: Untreated depression or stress.
   - Prevention: Seek professional help and build supportive relationships.

6. Stroke
   - Cause: High blood pressure, smoking, obesity.
   - Prevention: Manage blood pressure, eat healthily, and avoid smoking.

7. Erectile Dysfunction (ED)
   - Cause: Poor circulation, diabetes, stress.
   - Prevention: Maintain cardiovascular health and manage stress.

8. Liver Disease
   - Cause: excessive alcohol consumption, hepatitis infections, and obesity.
   - Prevention: Limit alcohol intake, get vaccinated against hepatitis A and B, maintain a healthy weight, and avoid risky behaviors like drug use.

Understanding Testosterone and Men's Health

Testosterone plays a significant role in a man's physical, mental, and emotional well-being. Low testosterone, often linked to aging or lifestyle factors, can lead to fatigue, weight gain, and diminished vitality.

Causes of Low Testosterone

- <u>Natural Aging</u>: Levels naturally decline after age 30.

- <u>Poor Diet</u>: Nutritional deficiencies and excess processed foods reduce testosterone production. High blood sugar and poor insulin sensitivity can suppress testosterone. Excess omega-6 fatty acids (e.g., from processed vegetables oils) may negatively affect testosterone levels.

- <u>Stress and Sleep Deprivation</u>: Chronic stress and lack of quality sleep disrupt hormone balance. High cortisol can lead to fatigue, weight gain, and mood changes, exacerbating testosterone decline. Testosterone is primarily produced during deep sleep, so insufficient or poor-quality sleep (less than 7 hours per night) reduces levels. Sleep disorders like sleep apnea can further disrupt hormone production.

- <u>Lack of Physical Activity</u>: A sedentary lifestyle reduces testosterone production, while regular exercise (especially weightlifting and high-intensity interval training) boosts it.

- <u>Obesity</u>: Fat cells convert testosterone into estrogen through a process called aromatization, leading to lower testosterone levels. Visceral fat (fat around the organs) is particularly detrimental to hormone balance.

- <u>Excessive Alcohol Consumption, Smoking and Drug Use</u>: Alcohol, particularly in large quantities, interferes with the testicles' ability to produce testosterone. Beer contains phytoestrogens from hops, which may further lower testosterone. Smoking damages blood vessels and reduces oxygen delivery, indirectly affecting testosterone production. Recreational drugs, such as anabolic steroids and opioids, can severely suppress testosterone.

- <u>Environmental Toxins</u>: Exposure to endocrine disruptors, such as bisphenol A (BPA) in plastics, phthalates, and pesticides, can interfere with testosterone production. Heavy metals like lead or mercury can also harm hormone health.

- <u>Medical Conditions</u>: Hypogonadism: A condition where the testes don't produce enough testosterone. Type 2 Diabetes: Poor insulin sensitivity is linked to lower testosterone levels. Thyroid Disorders: An underactive or overactive thyroid can affect hormone production. Chronic Illnesses: Kidney disease, liver disease, and HIV/AIDS can impair testosterone production. Inflammation: Chronic inflammation (e.g., from autoimmune diseases) negatively impacts hormone regulation.

Boosting Testosterone Naturally

- Eat a balanced diet rich in zinc, magnesium, and healthy fats.
- Exercise regularly, focusing on strength training, and maintain a healthy weight.
- Sleep 7–9 hours nightly to support hormone production.
- Reduce stress through mindfulness or relaxation techniques.
- Limit alcohol and avoid smoking.
- Minimize toxin exposure.

Practical Health Tips for Men

1. Prioritize Regular Checkups:

   Get annual physicals and screenings for blood pressure, cholesterol, blood sugar, and prostate health.

2. Adopt a Balanced Diet:

   Focus on lean proteins, whole grains, colorful vegetables, and healthy fats. Avoid processed foods, and reduce your intake of sugar, trans fats, and sugary drinks. Stay hydrated by drinking plenty of water daily to support metabolism and overall health.

3. Exercise Regularly:

   Combine strength training, cardio, and flexibility exercises to build a robust and resilient body.

4. Manage Stress Effectively:

   Practice mindfulness, maintain strong relationships, and create time for rest and renewal.

5. Sleep Well:

   Sleep is essential for hormone balance, mental clarity, and energy. Prioritize rest as part of your health routine.

Healthy Dieting is a Must!

Top 10 Healthiest Foods for Men

These foods are nutrient-dense and provide key nutrients that support men's overall health, including heart health, muscle building, and hormone balance.

1. Fatty fish (salmon, mackerel). **Benefits**: High in omega-3 fatty acids, which improve heart health, reduce inflammation, and support testosterone production
2. Leafy greens (spinach, kale, etc.). **Benefits**: Rich in magnesium, which supports muscle function, reduces inflammation and helps maintain healthy testosterone levels.
3. Eggs. **Benefits**: Provide protein, healthy fats, and cholesterol needed for testosterone production and muscle repair.

4. Berries (blueberries, raspberries, strawberries, blackberries). **Benefits:** Packed with antioxidants to combat oxidative stress and support brain and heart health.
5. Nuts and seeds (walnuts, almonds, pumpkin seeds). **Benefits:** High in healthy fats, zinc, and magnesium, which boost testosterone and improve cardiovascular health.
6. Whole grains (quinoa, oatmeal, long grain or brown rice). **Benefits:** Provide complex carbohydrates for sustained energy and fiber for heart and digestive health.
7. Lean meats (chicken, turkey). **Benefits:** High in protein and iron, which support muscle building and energy levels.
8. Legumes (lentils, chickpeas). **Benefits:** Packed with protein, fiber, and essential minerals like magnesium and zinc.
9. Garlic. **Benefits:** Contains allicin, which may lower cortisol levels and improve testosterone production.
10. Avocados. **Benefits:** High in monounsaturated fats, potassium, and vitamin B6, which support heart health and hormone balance.

Foods to Avoid

1. Sugary drinks (sodas, energy drinks, sweetened coffee drinks, etc.)
2. Processed meats (bacon, sausage, deli meats, etc.)
3. Trans fats (fried foods, margarine, packaged snacks)
4. Refined carbohydrates (white bread, pastries, sugary cereals)
5. Excessive alcohol (beer, liquor, sugary cocktails)
6. Highly processed snacks (frozen meals, chips, instant noodles, etc.)
7. Fried foods (such as fried chicken, French fries, onion rings, etc.)
8. Excessive Soy products (soy milk, tofu)

9. Artificial sweeteners (aspartame, saccharin (in diet sodas or sugar-free products))
10. High-sodium foods (canned soups, salty snacks, processed cheese)

Prostate Health and Aging Concerns

Prostate and urinary health are common concerns for men, particularly as they age. Regular screenings, including PSA tests, are essential to monitor prostate health and address potential issues early.

Key Takeaways for Men's Health and Wholeness

- Invest in Preventive Care: Take steps today to avoid chronic illnesses later.
- Small Habits Matter: Simple daily routines compound into long-term health benefits.
- Be Proactive: Don't ignore warning signs or delay medical care when needed.

Your health is an investment—not only for your body but also for your relationships, productivity, and spiritual well-being. By prioritizing your physical health, you are actively participating in God's plan for a life of abundance and purpose.

This chapter serves as a reminder that maintaining your health is not only a personal responsibility but also a demonstration of love for yourself and those who depend on you. True wholeness begins when you take charge of your well-being.

Chapter 2
The Man and His Money
Financial Health

What is Financial Health?

Financial health refers to the overall state of an individual's financial situation, encompassing their ability to manage money, meet current and future obligations, and achieve financial goals without undue stress. Just as physical health reflects how well our bodies function, financial health measures the stability, security, and resilience of our financial lives.

At its core, financial health is about balance and stewardship—using resources wisely to sustain and improve your quality of life while planning for the future. It's not merely about how much money you have; it's about how effectively you manage what you have.

7 Key Components of Financial Health:

1 | Income Stability

Income stability is consistently earning enough money to cover your basic needs (housing, food, transportation, etc.) and discretionary expenses. Income stability refers to having a reliable source of earnings that consistently meets your needs and allows for savings and investments.

Why It's Important:

A stable income is the foundation of financial health. It ensures that you can pay for necessities like housing, food, transportation, and healthcare while also funding discretionary spending and long-term goals.

How to Achieve It

- Secure steady employment or develop multiple income streams to reduce dependency on a single source.
- Build skills and pursue education or certifications to increase your earning potential.
- Plan for income diversification through side businesses, freelancing, or passive income sources.

2 | Spending Control

Spending control means practicing disciplined spending habits by living within your means by managing your expenses wisely and avoiding unnecessary debt or financial strain.

Why It's Important

Overspending leads to debt, which can quickly spiral out of control. Controlled spending ensures you maintain financial balance.

How to Achieve It

- Create and stick to a budget that categorizes your expenses (e.g., needs, wants, savings).
- Practice delayed gratification and prioritize needs over wants.
- Avoid impulse purchases and keep track of where your money goes.

3 | Savings and Investments

Savings and investments refers to having an emergency fund to handle unexpected expenses and making intentional investments to grow wealth over time.

Savings and investments ensure financial security in the short term and wealth growth in the long term.

Why It's Important

Savings provide a safety net for emergencies, while investments grow your wealth and help you achieve larger goals like retirement.

How to Achieve It:

- Build an emergency fund with at least 3–6 months' worth of living expenses.
- Open retirement accounts (e.g., 401(k), IRA) and invest consistently.
- Diversify investments (e.g., stocks, bonds, real estate) to reduce risk.
- Automate savings to make it a consistent habit.

4 | Debt Management

Debt management is keeping debt levels manageable by prioritizing repayment and avoiding high-interest debt that could lead to financial instability.

Debt management involves responsibly borrowing and repaying loans or credit to avoid financial strain.

Why It's Important

Excessive or mismanaged debt can derail your financial stability, limiting your ability to save and invest.

How to Achieve It

- Prioritize paying off high-interest debt (e.g., credit cards).

- Avoid unnecessary borrowing; only take on debt for meaningful purposes (e.g., a home or education).
- Use the snowball or avalanche method to tackle debt systematically.
- Regularly monitor your credit score and maintain good credit.

5 | Financial Planning

The basics of financial planning is setting clear short-term and long-term financial goals, such as saving for a home, retirement, or your children's education, and actively working toward achieving them. Financial planning is the process of setting clear goals and creating a roadmap to achieve them.

Why It's Important

Planning gives your finances direction, helping you stay focused on long-term objectives while managing short-term needs.

How to Achieve It

- Set SMART financial goals (Specific, Measurable, Achievable, Relevant, Time-bound).
- Work with a financial advisor if needed to develop strategies.
- Regularly review and adjust your financial plan as circumstances change.
- Incorporate milestones to celebrate progress and stay motivated.

6 | Insurance and Risk Management

Insurance and risk management protect you and your family from financial loss due to unexpected events. Protecting yourself and your loved ones with appropriate insurance coverage (health, life, auto, etc.) to mitigate risks and avoid financial crises.

Why It's Important

Emergencies like illness, accidents, or natural disasters can drain your finances. Insurance helps mitigate those risks.

How to Achieve It

- Ensure adequate coverage for health, life, auto, home, and disability insurance.
- Regularly review policies to ensure they meet your current needs.
- Build a separate fund for uncovered risks (e.g., deductibles, uncovered claims).

7 | Generosity and Stewardship

Incorporating tithing, giving, and philanthropy as part of your financial habits, which reflect trust in God's provision and a commitment to helping others.

Generosity and stewardship focus on using your financial resources to bless others and honor God.

Why It's Important

Giving fosters a spirit of gratitude and trust in God's provision, while stewardship ensures you manage your resources responsibly.

How to Achieve It

- Consistently tithe as an expression of faith and obedience to God. Give to causes and charities that align with your values.

- Budget for generosity, making giving a regular part of your financial plan.
- View yourself as a manager of God's resources, ensuring you use them wisely for His glory.

The Interconnection of Components

These components do not operate in isolation. For instance:

- Poor spending habits can lead to unmanageable debt, while lack of savings makes you vulnerable in emergencies.
- Without financial planning, it's challenging to achieve stability or wealth.
- Generosity without sound financial management can leave you struggling to meet your own needs.

Achieving financial health requires balancing these elements harmoniously to create a life of stability, peace, and purpose. It's not just about wealth but about thriving in every area of your financial life while honoring God and serving others.

The Biblical Perspective on Financial Health

The Bible provides timeless wisdom on managing money and maintaining financial health. Proverbs 21:5 says, *"The plans of the diligent lead surely to plenty, but those of everyone who is hasty, surely to poverty."* Financial health requires intentionality, patience, and diligence.

Additionally, 1 Timothy 6:10 reminds us that *"the love of money is the root of all evil,"* emphasizing that financial health is not about idolizing wealth but rather about using it responsibly as a tool for God's purposes. Stewardship is at the heart of financial well-being; everything we have belongs to God, and we are called to manage it wisely (Psalm 24:1).

Why Financial Health Matters

Financial health impacts nearly every aspect of your life. Poor financial health can lead to stress, strained relationships, and limited opportunities. Conversely, good financial health fosters peace of mind, freedom to pursue your passions, and the ability to bless others generously.

By cultivating financial health, you position yourself to live a balanced, prosperous, and God-honoring life, ensuring that your resources are a blessing rather than a burden.

Chapter 3

The Man and His Faith
Spiritual Health

"For what shall it profit a man, if he shall gain the whole world, and lose his own soul? Or what shall a man give in exchange for his soul?"
Mark 8:36-37

What is Spiritual Health?

Spiritual health refers to a state of harmony, purpose, and connection to God and His divine plan for your life. It encompasses your relationship with God, alignment with His will, and the depth of your faith. Spiritual health is not about religion or rituals alone; it is about cultivating a meaningful and intimate relationship with God, experiencing peace, joy, and strength that flows from that connection.

Just as physical health nurtures the body and mental health strengthens the mind, spiritual health nourishes the soul. It equips you to navigate life's challenges with hope, resilience, and a sense of eternal perspective. A spiritually healthy person lives with purpose, guided by God's Word, and seeks to reflect His love in every area of life.

Key Aspects of Spiritual Health

1. <u>Relationship with God</u>: Actively seeking a deeper connection with God through prayer, worship, and study of His Word.
2. <u>Faith and Trust</u>: Believing in God's promises, even in difficult circumstances, and trusting His plan for your life.

3. <u>Obedience to God's Will</u>: Aligning your life with God's principles and commands as revealed in Scripture.
4. <u>Love and Service:</u> Demonstrating God's love through acts of kindness, compassion, and service to others.
5. <u>Inner Peace</u>: Finding contentment and rest in God, regardless of external circumstances.

How to Obtain Spiritual Health

Achieving spiritual health is a journey that requires intentionality, discipline, and dependence on God's grace. Here's how to cultivate it:

1 | Commit to Daily Prayer and Communication with God

Why It's Important

Prayer is the foundation of spiritual health, fostering intimacy with God.

How to Practice

Set aside dedicated time each day to pray, whether in the morning, evening or throughout the day.

- Be honest and open in your prayers, expressing gratitude, seeking guidance, and confessing sins.
- Practice listening to God through silence and reflection.

2 | Study God's Word

Why It's Important

The Bible is God's revealed truth, offering guidance, encouragement, and correction.

How to Practice

- Read and meditate on Scripture daily, focusing on passages that speak to your current situation.
- Join a Bible study group to gain deeper insights and accountability.
- Memorize key verses to keep God's Word in your heart.

3 | Engage in Worship

Why It's Important

Worship draws you closer to God and reminds you of His greatness and love.

How to Practice

- Participate in corporate worship at church to connect with others and honor God collectively.
- Create a personal atmosphere of worship through music, gratitude, and reflection.
- Cultivate a lifestyle of worship by acknowledging God in all you do.

4 | Cultivate Fellowship with Believers

Why It's Important: Community strengthens faith, provides support, and fosters accountability.

How to Practice

- Attend church regularly and participate in small groups or ministries.

- Surround yourself with spiritually mature individuals who can mentor and encourage you.
- Be an active part of the body of Christ by serving others.

5 | Seek Holiness and Obedience

Why It's Important

Spiritual health thrives in purity and alignment with God's standards.

How to Practice

- Regularly examine your heart and repent of sin.
- Strive to live out biblical principles in your decisions, relationships, and lifestyle.
- Depend on the Holy Spirit to empower you for righteous living.

6 | Practice Gratitude and Contentment

Why It's Important

Gratitude shifts your focus from lack to abundance, fostering joy and trust in God.

How to Practice

- Keep a gratitude journal, noting daily blessings.
- Thank God in all circumstances, trusting His sovereignty.
- Reflect on His past faithfulness to build confidence in His future provision.

7 | Serve Others in Love

Why It's Important

Serving others demonstrates God's love and fulfills His command to love your neighbor.

How to Practice

- Volunteer in your community or church.
- Offer kindness and support to those in need.
- Pray for others and seek ways to bless them.

8 | Embrace Rest and Renewal

Why It's Important

Rest is essential for spiritual health, allowing you to reflect on God and rejuvenate your soul.

How to Practice

- Honor the Sabbath by dedicating time to worship and rest.
- Take regular breaks from busyness to reflect and recharge spiritually.
- Spend time in nature or quiet spaces to connect with God's creation.

The Benefits of Spiritual Health

When you prioritize spiritual health, you experience:

- Peace: A deep calm that surpasses understanding (Philippians 4:7).

- <u>Joy</u>: Fulfillment and happiness rooted in God's presence (Psalm 16:11).
- <u>Guidance</u>: Wisdom and direction from the Holy Spirit (John 16:13).
- <u>Strength</u>: Resilience to endure challenges with God's help (Isaiah 40:31).
- <u>Purpose</u>: Clarity about your God-given mission and calling (Jeremiah 29:11).

Spiritual health is the cornerstone of a fulfilling and purposeful life. By nurturing your relationship with God, embracing His truth, and living out your faith, you can walk in the abundant life He promises (John 10:10). It's a daily commitment, but the rewards—peace, joy, and eternal hope—are immeasurable.

Scriptures on Spiritual Health

Here are several scriptures that speak to the concept of spiritual health and its importance in maintaining a vibrant relationship with God:

1 | Spiritual Vitality and Connection with God

John 15:5: "I [Jesus] am the vine; you are the branches. If you remain in me and I in you, you will bear much fruit; apart from me you can do nothing."

This verse emphasizes the importance of staying connected to Jesus for spiritual growth and vitality.

Matthew 6:33: "But seek first his kingdom and his righteousness, and all these things will be given to you as well."

Prioritizing your relationship with God leads to overall well-being and fulfillment.

2 | Peace and Rest in God

Philippians 4:6-7: "Do not be anxious about anything, but in every situation, by prayer and petition, with thanksgiving, present your requests to God. And the peace of God, which transcends all understanding, will guard your hearts and your minds in Christ Jesus."

A spiritually healthy person experiences God's peace through prayer and trust.

Matthew 11:28-30: "Come to me, all you who are weary and burdened, and I will give you rest. Take my yoke upon you and learn from me, for I am gentle and humble in heart, and you will find rest for your souls. For my yoke is easy and my burden is light."

Rest for the soul comes from surrendering to Jesus and His guidance.

3 | Renewal and Transformation

Romans 12:2: "Do not conform to the pattern of this world, but be transformed by the renewing of your mind. Then you will be able to test and approve what God's will is—his good, pleasing and perfect will."

Spiritual health involves a transformed mind and life that align with God's will.

Isaiah 40:31: "But those who hope in the Lord will renew their strength. They will soar on wings like eagles; they will run and not grow weary, they will walk and not be faint."

Waiting on God and placing hope in Him brings spiritual renewal and strength.

4 | Spiritual Discipline

1 Timothy 4:7-8: "Have nothing to do with godless myths and old wives' tales; rather, train yourself to be godly. For physical training is of some value, but godliness has value for all things, holding promise for both the present life and the life to come."

Spiritual health requires discipline and consistent growth in godliness.

Joshua 1:8: "Keep this Book of the Law always on your lips; meditate on it day and night, so that you may be careful to do everything written in it. Then you will be prosperous and successful."

Regular meditation on God's Word leads to spiritual prosperity and success.

5 | Love and Service

1 Corinthians 13:13: "And now these three remain: faith, hope, and love. But the greatest of these is love."

Spiritual health is marked by love for God and others.

Galatians 5:22-23: "But the fruit of the Spirit is love, joy, peace, forbearance, kindness, goodness, faithfulness, gentleness and self-control. Against such things there is no law."

A spiritually healthy life bears the fruit of the Holy Spirit.

6 | Trust and Dependence on God

Proverbs 3:5-6: "Trust in the Lord with all your heart and lean not on your own understanding; in all your ways submit to him, and he will make your paths straight."

Spiritual health is rooted in total trust and dependence on God.

Psalm 23:1-3: "The Lord is my shepherd, I lack nothing. He makes me lie down in green pastures, he leads me beside quiet waters, he refreshes my soul. He guides me along the right paths for his name's sake."

God refreshes and restores the soul of those who follow Him.

7 | Spiritual Strength in Trials

2 Corinthians 12:9-10: "But he said to me, 'My grace is sufficient for you, for my power is made perfect in weakness.' Therefore I will boast all the more gladly about my weaknesses, so that Christ's power may rest on me."

Spiritual health is strengthened in dependence on God's grace during hardships.

James 1:2-4: "Consider it pure joy, my brothers and sisters, whenever you face trials of many kinds, because you know that the testing of your faith produces perseverance. Let perseverance finish its work so that you may be mature and complete, not lacking anything."

Trials develop spiritual maturity and completeness.

8 | Abundant Life in Christ

John 10:10: "The thief comes only to steal and kill and destroy; I have come that they may have life, and have it to the full."

True spiritual health comes from experiencing the abundant life Jesus offers.

Psalm 16:11: "You make known to me the path of life; you will fill me with joy in your presence, with eternal pleasures at your right hand."

Joy and fulfillment are found in God's presence.

These scriptures provide a solid foundation for understanding and pursuing spiritual health in every area of life.

Chapter 4
The Man and His Mind
Mental Health

Mental health is a cornerstone of holistic well-being, encompassing your emotional, psychological, and social stability. It affects how you think, feel, and behave, influencing your relationships, decision-making, and ability to navigate life's challenges. In a society that often glorifies busyness and external achievement, taking care of your mental health is an act of self-love and a critical step toward living the abundant life God intends for you.

The Importance of Mental Health

Just as the physical body needs care to function optimally, your mind requires attention and nurturing. Mental health impacts every facet of life:

- Spiritual Life: A troubled mind can hinder your ability to focus on prayer, worship, and meditation on God's Word.
- Relationships: Poor mental health can strain your interactions with others, creating misunderstandings and conflict.
- Productivity: A healthy mind enhances creativity, focus, and resilience, enabling you to fulfill your God-given purpose.

Neglecting mental health can lead to stress, anxiety, depression, and even physical illnesses. Conversely, prioritizing mental well-being enables you to flourish in your relationship with God, yourself, and others.

LOVE THYSELF

Mental Health and Loving Yourself

Jesus commanded us to love our neighbors as ourselves (Matthew 22:39). Embedded in this command is the understanding that self-love is foundational. Loving yourself means recognizing your worth as a child of God and caring for your mental, emotional, and physical health.

Caring for your mental health reflects good stewardship of the mind God has given you. Proverbs 4:23 reminds us, "Above all else, guard your heart, for everything you do flows from it." In biblical terms, the "heart" often represents the mind and emotions. Guarding your mental health is essential for living a purposeful and balanced life.

Biblical References on Mental Health

The Bible offers wisdom and encouragement for maintaining mental health:

Philippians 4:6-7: "Do not be anxious about anything, but in every situation, by prayer and petition, with thanksgiving, present your requests to God. And the peace of God, which transcends all understanding, will guard your hearts and your minds in Christ Jesus."

This verse encourages us to surrender our anxieties to God through prayer, finding peace and mental stability in His presence.

2 Timothy 1:7: "For the Spirit God gave us does not make us timid, but gives us power, love, and self-discipline."

God's Spirit empowers us to cultivate a sound mind and reject fear.

Isaiah 26:3: "You will keep in perfect peace those whose minds are steadfast, because they trust in you."

Trusting in God fosters peace and stability in our thoughts.

Psalm 34:18: "The Lord is close to the brokenhearted and saves those who are crushed in spirit."

God's nearness offers hope and comfort in times of mental and emotional struggle.

Practical Tools for Maintaining Mental Health

1. Renew Your Mind

    Romans 12:2: *"Do not conform to the pattern of this world, but be transformed by the renewing of your mind."* Replace negative or destructive thought patterns with God's truth. Practice affirmations based on Scripture, such as declaring, "I am fearfully and wonderfully made" (Psalm 139:14).

2. Practice Gratitude

    Gratitude shifts your focus from lack to abundance, fostering a positive mindset. Keep a gratitude journal, listing daily blessings and answered prayers.

3. Engage in Rest and Sabbath

    Mental health requires rest. Jesus modeled the importance of withdrawing to quiet places for renewal (Mark 6:31). Prioritize sleep, relaxation, and Sabbath observance to recharge your mind.

4. Seek Community

   Proverbs 27:17 says, *"As iron sharpens iron, so one person sharpens another."* Surround yourself with supportive, godly friends who encourage and uplift you.

5. Set Healthy Boundaries

   Protect your mental health by setting boundaries in relationships, work, and commitments. Learn to say no when necessary to avoid burnout.

6. Engage in Professional Support

   There's no shame in seeking help from counselors, therapists, or mental health professionals. Proverbs 11:14 reminds us that "where there is no guidance, a people falls, but in an abundance of counselors there is safety."

7. Stay Physically Active

   Exercise improves mental clarity, reduces stress, and releases endorphins that enhance mood. 1 Corinthians 6:19 reminds us that our bodies are temples of the Holy Spirit—caring for your physical health also supports mental well-being.

8. Cultivate a Prayer and Meditation Routine

   Spend time in God's presence, meditating on His Word and listening for His voice. This brings peace and centers your thoughts on His promises.

Benefits of Being Mentally Healthy

1. Peace of Mind

   A mentally healthy person experiences God's peace, even amidst challenges (Philippians 4:7).

2. Improved Relationships

   Mental stability enhances communication, empathy, and the ability to build healthy connections.

3. Increased Productivity

   A clear mind allows for better focus, creativity, and problem-solving abilities.

4. Emotional Resilience

   Mentally healthy individuals can navigate stress and setbacks with grace and confidence.

5. Closer Relationship with God

   A healthy mind fosters deeper engagement in prayer, worship, and Scripture study.

Conclusion

Your mental health is a gift from God and a vital part of loving yourself. By nurturing your mind with biblical truths, healthy practices, and God's peace, you position yourself to live a balanced and fulfilling life. Remember, loving yourself isn't selfish—it's stewardship. As you care for your mental health, you honor God, enhance your relationships, and empower yourself to serve His kingdom effectively. Be encouraged to take intentional steps toward mental wholeness, trusting that God's Spirit will guide and sustain you every step of the way.

Chapter 5
The Man and His Family
Family Health

Family health is essential to living a fulfilling and balanced life. The family unit, as designed by God, serves as the foundation of society and the first place where love, support, and purpose are cultivated. A healthy family nurtures every member's spiritual, emotional, and relational well-being, fostering unity and stability that honors God and strengthens individuals.

The Importance of Family Health

Family health encompasses the dynamics, relationships, and overall functioning of the family unit. It is critical in shaping identity, values, and emotional stability. A healthy family provides:

- Emotional Support: A safe space where members feel loved, valued, and understood.
- Spiritual Growth: A foundation for teaching and living out biblical principles.
- Relational Stability: Strong bonds that build trust and resilience during challenges.
- Legacy: A generational impact that reflects God's love and purposes.

When families are healthy, individuals thrive, and communities grow stronger. Conversely, when family health is neglected, the effects can ripple into spiritual, mental, and relational struggles.

The Biblical Structure of the Family Unit

God designed the family to reflect His order and love. Scripture provides a clear blueprint for the roles and responsibilities within a family:

LOVE THYSELF

The Husband and Father

The man's role as husband and father is foundational to the health of the family. He is called to be the household's spiritual leader, provider, and protector.

- <u>Spiritual Leader</u>: The husband is tasked with leading his family in faith. *"Husbands, love your wives, just as Christ loved the church and gave himself up for her"* (Ephesians 5:25). His leadership should be marked by love, humility, and a Christlike example.
- <u>Provider</u>: *"Anyone who does not provide for their relatives, and especially for their own household, has denied the faith and is worse than an unbeliever"* (1 Timothy 5:8). Providing isn't just financial; it includes emotional and spiritual provision as well.
- <u>Protector</u>: The father is called to protect his family physically and spiritually, guarding them from harm and leading them in God's ways.

The Wife and Mother

The wife and mother play a vital role in nurturing and managing the home.

- <u>Supportive Partner</u>: *"The Lord God said, 'It is not good for the man to be alone. I will make a helper suitable for him'"* (Genesis 2:18). She is a partner in fulfilling God's purpose for the family.
- <u>Nurturer</u>: Mothers have a unique role in shaping children's character and faith through love and teaching (Proverbs 31:26-28).

The Children

Children are a blessing from God (Psalm 127:3) and are called to honor and obey their parents.

- Obedience: *"Children, obey your parents in the Lord, for this is right"* (Ephesians 6:1).
- Honor: *"Honor your father and mother"* (Exodus 20:12). Respecting parental guidance is key to a healthy family dynamic.

Family Health and Loving Yourself

Loving yourself includes honoring the roles and relationships God has placed in your family. A healthy family dynamic fosters self-esteem, purpose, and emotional security, which are vital aspects of self-love. When you contribute to a healthy family environment, you reflect God's love and care, which in turn nurtures your own well-being.

Biblical References on Family Health

Joshua 24:15: *"But as for me and my household, we will serve the Lord."* Families that prioritize God create a foundation of spiritual health.

Colossians 3:13: *"Bear with each other and forgive one another if any of you has a grievance against someone. Forgive as the Lord forgave you."* Forgiveness and patience are key to maintaining harmony in the family.

Proverbs 22:6: *"Start children off on the way they should go, and even when they are old they will not turn from it."* Spiritual training of children is a vital responsibility of the family.

1 Corinthians 13:4-7: *"Love is patient, love is kind. It does not envy, it does not boast, it is not proud."* This passage highlights the attitudes that should define all family relationships.

Practical Tools for Maintaining Family Health

1. Establish Family Devotions: Set aside regular time for prayer, Bible reading, and worship as a family.

2. Communicate Openly: Encourage honest and respectful conversations. Make it safe for family members to express their thoughts and feelings.

3. Prioritize Quality Time: Spend intentional time together, whether through shared meals, activities, or family traditions.

4. Practice Forgiveness and Grace: Address conflicts quickly and seek reconciliation, embodying Christ's love and forgiveness.

5. Set Boundaries: Establish rules and expectations that promote respect, accountability, and balance within the home.

6. Model Christlike Behavior: Demonstrate love, patience, humility, and faithfulness in your daily interactions.

7. Encourage Growth and Learning: Support each family member's individual talents and encourage personal and spiritual development.

8. Serve Together: Engage in acts of service as a family, reinforcing values of generosity and compassion.

Benefits of a Healthy Family Unit

1. Stronger Relationships: Healthy families enjoy deeper bonds and greater trust among members.

2. Spiritual Growth: A spiritually centered family creates an environment where faith thrives.

3. <u>Emotional Stability</u>: A supportive family provides security and resilience during difficult times.

4. <u>Generational Legacy</u>: Healthy families leave a lasting impact on future generations, modeling God's love and principles.

5. <u>Joy and Fulfillment</u>: Families that prioritize health experience greater joy, unity, and satisfaction in their relationships.

Family health is a reflection of God's divine design for relationships. By nurturing your family's well-being, you honor God and contribute to your own personal growth and fulfillment. Healthy families are a testimony to God's love, providing a legacy of faith and purpose for generations to come. Take intentional steps to cultivate a thriving family unit, trusting God's guidance and strength to lead you. In doing so, you fulfill His command to love one another deeply and reflect His glory in your home.

Chapter 6
The Whole Man: A Pillar of Health in the Community

"Thou shalt love thy neighbor as thyself."
— Mark 12:31

The Power of a Whole Man in a Broken World

A man who is whole—physically, emotionally, mentally, and spiritually—is a transformative force in his community. When a man invests in his own well-being, he becomes a pillar of stability, strength, and hope, especially in communities plagued by gun violence, trauma, and systemic challenges. His wholeness creates a ripple effect that inspires others to heal, grow, and thrive.

In this chapter, we explore how a man's wholeness equips him to address the challenges in his community, offering solutions, leadership, and restoration to those who need it most.

The Impact of Wholeness on Community Health

1 | Modeling Resilience and Healing

A man who has worked through his own pain and trauma demonstrates that healing is possible. He becomes a living example that brokenness does not have to be permanent.

- <u>Resilience as a Testimony</u>: By overcoming personal struggles, he inspires others to confront and overcome their own.
- <u>Healing Through Leadership</u>: His emotional stability allows him to lead initiatives that promote mental health, conflict resolution, and community restoration.

2 | Building Trust and Connection

A whole man understands the importance of relationships. He becomes a bridge-builder in his community, fostering unity among diverse groups.

- Restoring Community Bonds: He actively connects with young men, families, and community leaders to create networks of support.
- Earning Trust Through Integrity: His consistent actions and character rebuild trust in areas where it has been broken by violence and systemic oppression.

3 | Addressing Trauma with Compassion

A man who has learned to love himself understands the pain of others. He brings compassion and empathy to his community, addressing the root causes of violence and trauma.

- Advocating for Mental Health Resources: He pushes for counseling services, trauma-informed care, and safe spaces for healing.
- Mentorship and Guidance: He steps into the lives of young men who are at risk, showing them a path toward purpose and wholeness.

The Whole Man's Role in a Community Plagued by Violence

Communities struggling with gun violence and trauma often lack visible examples of hope and leadership. A whole man can transform this narrative through intentional action and service.

THE WHOLE MAN: A PILLAR OF HEALTH IN THE COMMUNITY

1. Preventing Violence Through Presence

A whole man understands that violence often stems from unaddressed pain and unmet needs. His presence alone can de-escalate tensions and prevent conflicts.

- Being a Mediator: He steps into heated situations, offering wisdom and solutions instead of retaliation.
- Creating Safe Spaces: He helps establish community centers, mentorship programs, and recreational activities to keep youth engaged and away from harmful environments.

2. Promoting Education and Opportunity

Education and economic empowerment are essential to breaking cycles of violence. A whole man invests his time and resources into creating opportunities for his community.

- Advocating for Education: He supports schools, tutoring programs, and scholarships for young men and women.
- Building Career Pathways: He partners with local businesses and organizations to provide job training and employment opportunities.

3. Addressing the Root Causes of Trauma

Gun violence and community trauma are symptoms of deeper issues like poverty, systemic racism, and family breakdown. A whole man addresses these root causes with strategic action.

- Advocating for Social Justice: He works to reform systems that perpetuate inequality, such as policing, housing, and healthcare.

- Strengthening Families: He mentors fathers and husbands, helping them rebuild strong and stable homes that nurture children.

Practical Ways to Contribute to Community Health

A man who is whole doesn't just talk about change—he becomes the change. Here are some practical ways a whole man can contribute to the health of his community:

1. Mentorship Programs: Start or support initiatives that connect at-risk youth with mentors who provide guidance, accountability, and encouragement.
2. Community Advocacy: Use your voice to advocate for policies and programs that address violence, poverty, and inequality. Attend town halls, join advisory boards, and collaborate with local leaders.
3. Healing Circles: Organize or participate in safe spaces where men can share their experiences, process trauma, and find support.
4. Conflict Resolution Training: Equip yourself and others with tools to resolve disputes peacefully. Offer workshops on de-escalation and non-violent communication.
5. Volunteerism: Give your time to community centers, schools, shelters, and organizations that serve vulnerable populations.
6. Economic Empowerment: Invest in local businesses, teach financial literacy, and create pathways to entrepreneurship for young men and women.

A Vision for Community Wholeness

When men are whole, their communities reflect their health. Imagine a neighborhood where:

- Violence is replaced with mentorship and opportunity.
- Trauma is addressed through counseling and support systems.
- Families are strengthened, creating a foundation for future generations.

This vision is not a fantasy—it is achievable when men choose to love themselves enough to pour that same love into others.

The Spiritual Mandate to Heal the Broken

Loving your neighbor begins with loving yourself. Jesus' command to "love thy neighbor as thyself" (Mark 12:31) implies that self-love is the foundation of community love. A man who is whole recognizes that his healing is not just for him—it's a gift to be shared with others.

- Prayer and Intercession: A whole man stands in the gap for his community, lifting up its struggles and needs in prayer.
- Service and Sacrifice: He embraces a life of service, putting the needs of others before his own comfort.
- Spiritual Leadership: He leads by example, showing others how to live with integrity, faith, and purpose.

Key Takeaways:
Becoming a Whole Man for Your Community

1. Heal Yourself First: You cannot pour from an empty cup. Your own wholeness is essential to serving others effectively.
2. Invest in Relationships: Build trust and connection with those around you, especially the youth who look up to you.
3. Take Action: Don't wait for someone else to fix the

problems—be the change you want to see.

4. <u>Walk in Faith</u>: Lean on God for guidance and strength as you serve your community.

A whole man doesn't just survive—he thrives. And as he thrives, he lifts others with him. By loving yourself enough to become whole, you answer the call to love your neighbor and transform your community into a place of hope, healing, and restoration.

Closing Reflection

When a man steps into his wholeness, he becomes a reflection of God's love, a beacon of hope in dark places. Loving yourself is not just about personal fulfillment; it is the starting point for healing a broken world. Your wholeness can be the catalyst for a community's restoration. Will you answer the call?

Conclusion
Be Made Whole

A Man's Wholeness

The journey to love thyself is, at its core, the pursuit of wholeness. It is about embracing the divine design God has for your life and aligning every facet of your being—physical, spiritual, mental, financial, and family—to reflect His glory. Wholeness is not perfection; it is a state of harmony where each part of your life complements the other, creating a balanced and fulfilling existence.

As men, we are called to live with intentionality and purpose. God has equipped us to lead, to nurture, and to thrive. But to fulfill this calling, we must first be whole. Loving yourself isn't selfish; it is the stewardship of the life, gifts, and responsibilities entrusted to you by God. A man who loves himself understands his worth in Christ and lives from a place of strength, confidence, and grace.

Physical Wholeness

Your body is a temple of the Holy Spirit (1 Corinthians 6:19). Caring for it through proper nutrition, exercise, rest, and discipline is an act of worship. Physical health equips you to fulfill your God-given assignments with energy and endurance. Neglecting your body not only hinders your purpose but also diminishes the quality of life God intends for you.

By loving yourself physically, you demonstrate gratitude for the vessel God has given you. Your body becomes a reflection of His strength and care, enabling you to lead and serve effectively.

Spiritual Wholeness

At the core of every man's life is his relationship with God. Spiritual health is the foundation upon which all other areas are built. It is the source of wisdom, strength, and direction. Jesus' call to abide in Him (John 15:5) reminds us that without Him, we can do nothing.

A spiritually whole man prioritizes prayer, worship, and the study of God's Word. He leads his family in faith, seeks God's will in every decision, and walks in humility and obedience. This connection to God anchors his life, providing peace and purpose in every season.

Mental Wholeness

Your mind is a battlefield, and mental health is essential to living victoriously. The Apostle Paul reminds us to "be transformed by the renewing of your mind" (Romans 12:2). Mental wholeness requires guarding your thoughts, cultivating gratitude, and aligning your mindset with God's truth.

A mentally whole man is resilient, able to navigate stress, challenges, and setbacks with confidence. He seeks support when needed, practices self-care, and remains steadfast in the face of adversity. Loving yourself mentally means embracing the peace of God, which surpasses all understanding (Philippians 4:7).

Financial Wholeness

God calls us to be good stewards of the resources He provides. Financial wholeness involves managing money wisely, living within your means, and being generous. Proverbs 21:5 reminds us, "The plans of the diligent lead surely to abundance, but everyone who is hasty comes only to poverty."

A financially whole man understands that money is a tool, not an idol. He prioritizes planning, saving, and giving, ensuring that his resources are a blessing to his family, community, and God's kingdom. Financial health reduces stress, fosters stability, and allows you to live with integrity and purpose.

Family Wholeness

The family is a reflection of God's design for love and unity. A man's role as husband and father is pivotal to the health of the family unit. Ephesians 5:25 calls husbands to "love your wives, just as Christ loved the church and gave himself up for her." This sacrificial love fosters trust, respect, and harmony.

A whole man leads his family with humility, nurtures his children with wisdom, and cultivates an environment of love and support. He prioritizes relationships, communicates openly, and models godly character. Loving yourself as a family man means investing in the people God has entrusted to your care, building a legacy that honors Him.

The Benefits of Wholeness

A man who is whole—physically, spiritually, mentally, financially, and within his family—lives a life of balance and purpose. He is equipped to:

- Serve God Faithfully: Wholeness enables you to fully embrace your calling and live a life that glorifies God.
- Love Others Fully: A whole man can love his family, friends, and community without reservation or depletion.
- Navigate Challenges Resiliently: Wholeness provides the strength and wisdom to face life's storms with confidence.
- Build a Lasting Legacy: Your wholeness impacts not only your life but also future generations, leaving a

legacy of faith, love, and stability.

A Call to Action

The journey to wholeness requires intentionality, discipline, and grace. It begins with a decision to love yourself as God loves you. Commit to the daily practices that nurture your physical, spiritual, mental, financial, and family health. Seek God's guidance and rely on His strength to transform every area of your life.

Remember, wholeness is not achieved overnight. It is a lifelong journey of growth and refinement. Celebrate your progress, embrace God's grace in your imperfections, and remain steadfast in your pursuit of the abundant life He has promised (John 10:10).

As you close this chapter, take a moment to reflect on the steps you've taken and the commitments you're ready to make. Wholeness is within your reach, and with God's help, you can live a life that honors Him, blesses others, and fulfills your divine purpose. Love yourself well, and in doing so, glorify the One who made you whole.

ABOUT THE AUTHOR

Antonio M. Palmer

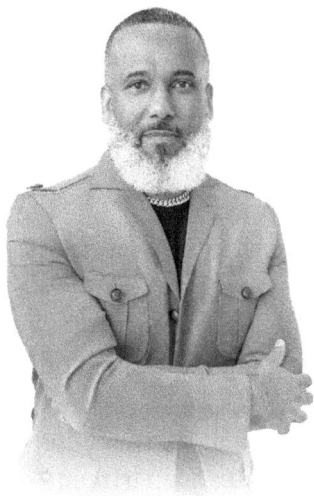

Bishop Antonio M. Palmer is the Senior Pastor of Kingdom Celebration Center and the Presiding Bishop of Kingdom Alliance of Churches International, overseeing a global network of 74 churches. With a ministry rooted in the Gospel since 1993, he planted his first church in Annapolis, Maryland, in 1995 and has since become a beacon of leadership, service, and transformation.

A passionate advocate for missions, Bishop Palmer leads leadership conferences, plants churches, and provides humanitarian aid to thousands of children in need across the globe. His work includes substantial financial support for orphanages in India and East Africa, demonstrating a steadfast commitment to serving the underserved.

A respected community leader, Bishop Palmer is celebrated for fostering unity and collaboration among diverse groups. His efforts focus on addressing critical issues, promoting meaningful dialogue, and inspiring transformative change. He holds a Bachelor of Divinity and a Master's in Pastoral Counseling and has been recognized with numerous accolades, including two Governor Citations, two County Executive Citations, and the prestigious Martin Luther King Jr. Drum Major Award.

Bishop Palmer's leadership extends beyond the pulpit. He has served as President of the United Black Clergy of Anne

Arundel County and as a community representative for the Severn Intergenerational Center. He serves on the Community Action Agency Board and has been a member of the United Way of Central Maryland RUN Board. His extensive collaboration with the County Executive's Office and community partners has focused on social justice, violence interruption, and equity.

Key Highlights of Bishop Palmer's Work:

- Advisor to the County Recovery Workgroup.
- Partnered with the Caucus of African American Leaders to advocate for media equity.
- Organized the "1000 Men March," a peaceful protest against racism that united 26 civic organizations and elected officials.
- Led COVID-19 response efforts through partnerships with the Anne Arundel County Health Department, including organizing testing sites and running remote learning programs for underserved communities.
- Oversees a food distribution program that serves over 1,000 individuals weekly.

As an entrepreneur, Bishop Palmer owns **Kingdom Publishing LLC**, **Antonio Marlin Art**, and **Kingdom Kare, Inc.**, a thriving nonprofit organization. He is also the author of six impactful books and two workbooks with teacher manuals:

Books
- *Love Thyself: Empowering Men for Healthy Living*
- *God's Rest Revealed: A Life Flowing with Milk and Honey*
- *Building an Effective Prayer Life*
- *Mark the Perfect Man: How to Find a Model of Maturity*
- *Revival: God Will Come Where You Are*
- *Little Kairo Conquers the World (Children's Book)*

Workbooks
- *Introductory to Spiritual Warfare*
- *Living By the Spirit*

Bishop Palmer's ministry is enriched by the love and partnership of his wife of 31 years, Dr. Barbara Palmer. Together, they share a legacy of faith, wisdom, and joy with their son Randy, daughter-in-law Kimberly, and five cherished grandchildren.

Author's contact information:

Email:

apalmerkcc@gmail.com
bishopkccodenton@gmail.com
apalmer@kingdomkareinc.com

Websites:

Artwork: https://antoniomarlin.art
Publishing: www.mykingdompublishing.com
Church: www.kingdomcelebrationcenter.com
Kingdom Kare, Inc: www.kingdomkareinc.com

www.ingramcontent.com/pod-product-compliance
Lightning Source LLC
Chambersburg PA
CBHW060258030426
42335CB00014B/1766